ALZHEIMER'S AND DEMENTIA:
HOW TO REDUCE THE RISKS OF
ALZHEIMER'S AND WAYS TO IMPROVE
THE QUALITY OF LIFE

IS DEMENTIA, AND ALZHEIMER'S DUE TO BRAIN INJURY, NUTRITIONAL DEFICIENCIES, INACTIVITY, OR SUBSTANCE ABUSE?
CAN THE NO SALT DIET CAUSE MEMORY LOSS MIMICKING ALZHEIMER'S DISEASE?

WHY SOME PEOPLE LIVE A LONG HEALTHY LIFE AND OTHERS GET ALZHEIMER'S

BY. S.ELIA

© 2018 BY S. ELIA ALL RIGHTS RESERVED

Self published by S.ELIA
Published by kindle direct publishing,
amazon.com

Disclaimer: this book is for information only and is not indented for diagnosis or treatments for any of the conditions mentioned.
For proper diagnosis and treatment consult your trusted doctor, and if in doubt get a second opinion OR EVEN A THIRD. Your health is the most precious thing you have, make sure you take care of yourself and your health.

S.ELIA
AUTHOR

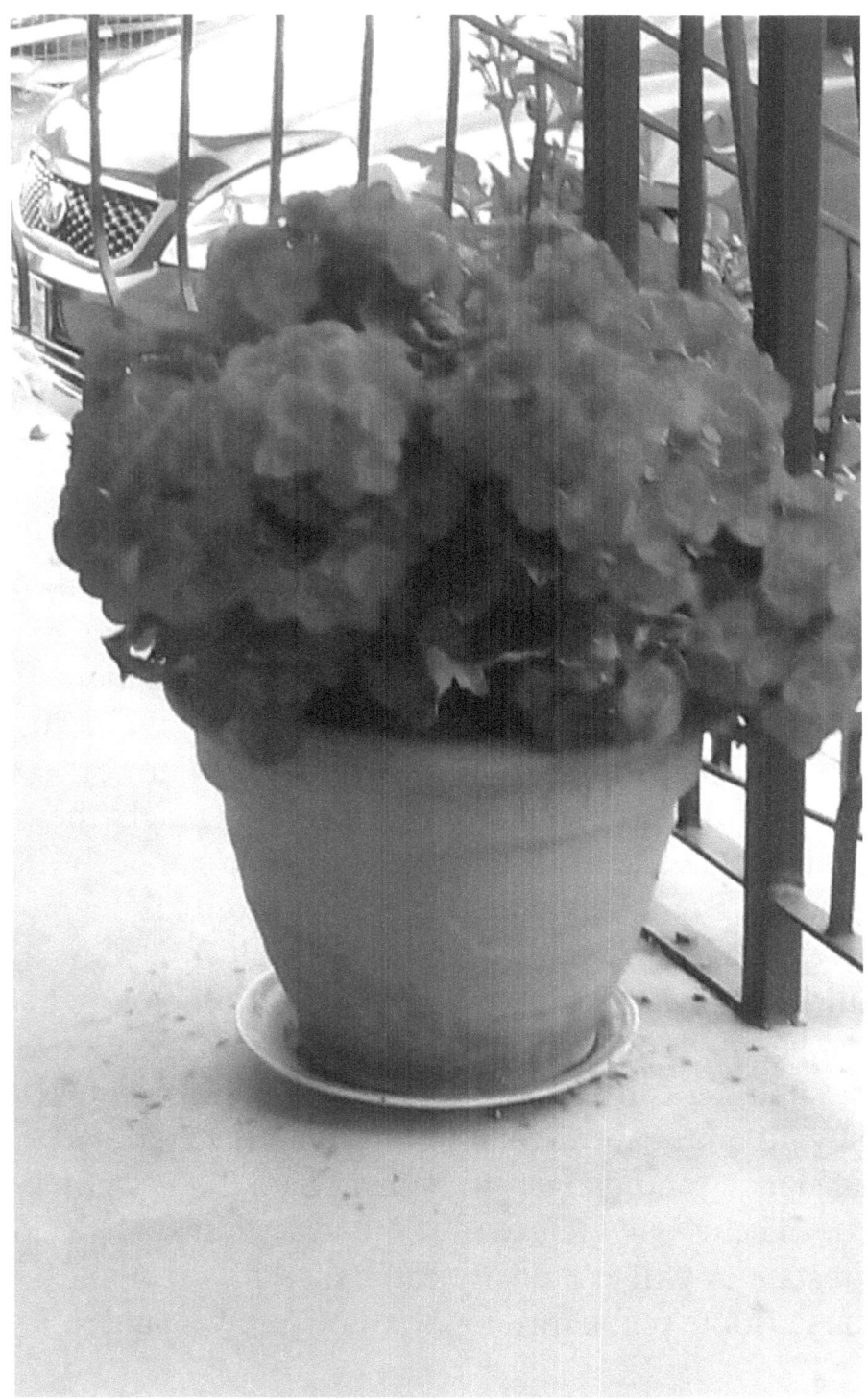

PROLOGUE

We all know that some day eventually we will die and we understand that, nobody can live for ever. However the quality of life we will live until that time comes is what it counts. some people will live a long healthy life and others will have minor or major health problems even before they reach the golden ripe age of 100 years old.. That can be genetic , from the genes one inherits from his parents, or from some other cause such as nutritional or pathology. When people are young and healthy they think they are on top of the world and nothing can do harm to them or their body and they go on to abuse their bodies with dangerous substances and dangerous stunts. Sadly that's not true .The use and abuse of some dangerous substances will eventually catch up with them and cause some real harm to their body, brain and

mind with mild or severe symptoms. of course that's not always the case but it does happen. Abusing their body with dangerous substances and a lack of proper nutrition can age people years before their normal aging .
. The way people live when they are young, can have an effect on their health and the risk to get dementia in the future. The choices you make over the course of any average day , smoking, using drugs, poor diets leading to nutritional deficiencies, can determine whether you'll develop dementia years from now, as well as how quickly the disease will progress . So it is important to know the risks factors. Prevention should start early to protect them from the ravaging effects of dementia when they reach their golden years.

On the other hand when people take good care of their bodies and have good nutrition in their diets, they can have a good healthy life and live their golden years without major health problems . We can see that in a few places of the world that people take care of themselves, eat right and keep busy and in those places Senility, dementia or Alzheimer is almost not existent.
There are about five such places on earth with top place the Japanese island Okinawa where the people tend their gardens
 for exercise and have good nutritional diet, and

remain healthy into very old age with few age related diseases.
The other four places where people live longer over 100 years old are, Sardinia, Italy, Loma Linda California, Nicoya, Costa Rica and Icaria Greece. The common element for their longevity in these places is their good nutritional diet and walking and exercises.
This might be a good prescription for all people that they want to live a long healthy life. The old adage take care of your body and your body will take care of your brain and mind which the ancient Greeks used to say " νους υγιης εν σοματι υγιη» is still as valid today, as it was thousands of years ago. .
Apparently the Greeks new one thing or two about taking care of both their bodies and their mind.

WHAT IS SENILITY AND DEMENTIA

Senility used to be considered as part of aging and was called senile dementia with serious mental and psychological problems. People used to believe that it was a normal part of aging and that was expected to happen with age. Now health professionals know better.

Dementia is not a specific disease but rather a term that describes a group of symptoms associated with the decline of memory and other skills that incapacitate that person to perform his daily activities. There are many conditions that cause the symptoms of senility and dementia, among them pathologies caused by vascular accidents to the brain after a stroke and Alzheimer's disease which has no clear cause. Any injury to the brain has the potential to cause serious damage and cause a decline to mental capacities of the patient.

WHAT IS ALZHEIMER DISEASE

Alzheimer's is a degenerative disease of the brain

with plagues scar formation in the brain interfering with the normal communication between the neuron of the brain.

Alzheimer's is the most common cause of dementia with memory loss and other cognitive abilities that interfere with daily life. Alzheimer's disease accounts for 60 percent of dementia cases. Alzheimer's disease is irreversible and destroys brain cells, causing thinking ability and memory to deteriorate

As the disease progresses it leads to increasingly severe problems to the functions of the brain. The most pronounced effects are memory loss which gets worse with time, confusion about events, times and places, disorientation mood and behavior changes. The disease eventually makes the patient incapable to care for himself and can easily get lost in familiar places. In advance stages of the disease the patient can't even recognize his family or friends, even their own name.

In any brain injury or damage to its parts there is loss of function in that particular part of the brain and the loss of communications between the damaged brain, the other parts of the brain and the parts of the body that is controlled by the damaged brain. If the brain damage is severe and extensive death is inevitable. In the case of Alzheimer's disease the damage to the brain is gradual with plaques formed all over the brain disrupting the communications between the parts of the brain and eventually shrink to a fraction of its original size due to the destruction of many neurons .

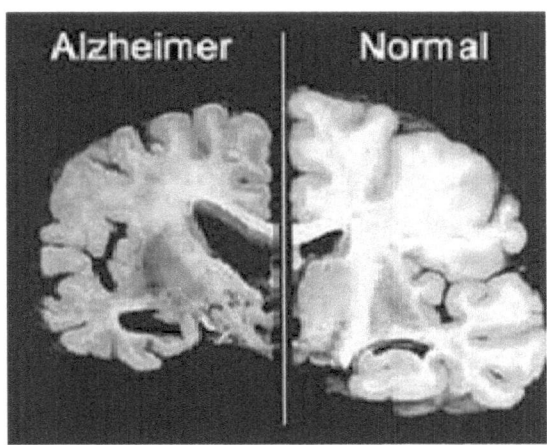

normal brain on the right side and abnormal atrophied brain on the left due to Alzheimer's desease.

As we ca see the brain affected by the Alzheimer's disease on the left have shrunk considerably to the healthy brain on the right. The question remains why? Is it due to a disease that killed the brain cells or is it a possibility that the brain was starved to death due to a lack of enough water in the cerebrospinal fluid that surrounds , bathe and protect the brain from any injury? In recent years there is a lot of talk about

a condition where the cerebrospinal fluid leaks out from the brain through the nose for unknown yet reasons and it has a salty taste. If enough cerebrospinal fluid leaks out, one can presume that the brain is left without enough protection and vulnerable to dehydration and injury .I think it is worth exploring that possibility and all patients exhibiting memory loss and other signs and symptoms of Alzheimer's disease to investigate if such a
Cerebrospinal fluid leak exists and correct it. There are doctors specializing in correcting this condition. The reasoning behind this idea, is that any wet substance when it looses its water it shrinks. The possibility exist when there is enough leakage of cerebrospinal fluid over a long period of time for the brain to starve of water and shrink . This might be a wild goose chase, but I think it is worth exploring. Anyway we leave that to the experts that do research for the causes of this dreadful disease and if they think that the shrinkage of the brain is due to the leakage of the cerebrospinal fluid , they will recommend the necessary correction.

HISTORY OF DEMENTIA AND ALZHEIMER

There was senility, dementia and Alzheimer's disease long before it was first described by Alois Alzheimer in 1906. He examined post mortem brains affected by dementia and published his findings, and from that time the disease was named after him in 1910. At that time he believed that senility dementia as it was called then, was the result of atherosclerosis, a common arterial disease that affects the human arteries with cholesterol deposit plaques obstructing the blood flow to the brain.

Alzheimer's is the most common cause of dementia with memory loss and other cognitive abilities serious enough to interfere with daily life. The greatest risk factor is increasing age, and the majority of people with Alzheimer's are 65 and older.

The early signs of dementia and Alzheimer is the loss of short memory where the patient does not remember recent events.

As the disease progresses the condition of the patient deteriorates until he or she is completely incapacitated.

Every year governments and other organizations spend millions of dollars in search of a cause, diagnosis and treatments for the disease. Despite all their efforts and the millions of dollars spent they still have not come up with a definite way what really causes the disease, or how to diagnose it properly, or an effective treatment. The only definite diagnosis is done after the patient dies and do a microscopic examination of the patient's brain.

It used to be considered a disease of old people usually over 65, but in rare occasions younger people can be affected too. Now they diagnose people with symptoms of Alzheimer's disease that are a lot younger. The youngest person ever diagnosed with dementia Alzheimer's disease was 27 years old. Maybe there are more younger people with this disease and they are not diagnosed yet due to their age. But the real question is, was that a real Alzheimer's disease or something else like a disease caused by nutritional deficiencies or some substance abuse. There are after all halusogenicc drugs, foods and plants that when consumed ,can cause or mimic the symptoms of dementia and Alzheimer's disease.

CAUSES OF DEMENTIA AND

ALZHEIMER'S.

The cause of dementia and Alzheimer's disease is anybody's guess. There are many theories and speculations about the cause of senility , dementia and Alzheimer's disease, but still there is no real provable cause.
Some scientists believe that the Alzheimer's disease is caused by a combination of genetic, lifestyle and environmental factors that affect the brain over time. However less than 5 percent is caused by genetic predisposition and the rest due to other causes.
It is very difficult to know for sure if the patient has the real life changing degenerative encephalopathy disease or something else caused by lifestyle or environmental factors which might be treatable or not, by changing the lifestyle or the environment.
It is a good idea to examine such factors or conditions in the hope that the patient can have a chance to get help with his condition if it is not the degenerative encephalopathy. As all scientist know the original main reason for suspecting that the patient has Alzheimer's disease is the memory loss. But there are a lot of reasons that a patient can have memory loss without having the deadly disease. Later on , We are going to examine such reasons that cause memory loss to humans, so that

we explore all possibilities with the hope that the patient can be diagnosed and properly treated if it is not the degenerative encephalopathy of Alzheimer's disease.

There are some studies that suggest that Alzheimer's runs in families and if one of the parents have Alzheimer's there is a chance their kids will inherit the disease. There is a debate in the scientific community, if it is inherited from the father or the mother, with some suggesting that the chances of **inheriting** it from your **mother** are higher than from your **father**. It seems that it is anybody's guess at the moment with some even doubting that it is inherited from either of parents.

There are theories and suggestions that smoked meats that contain nitrosamines, cause the liver to produce some fats that are toxic to the brain.
Even beer, cured meats, some cheeses, dry milk , fruits and vegetables, cosmetics, pesticides, tobacco products, rubber products balloons etc contain nitrosamines . makes you wonder if there is anything that is not causing dementia and Alzheimer .

The aluminum cooking utensils are also mentioned as a possible cause. And the list goes on and on.......... As long as we do not have a definite provable cause, meaning that if you remove the cause the patient will be cured, or you duplicate the disease in the laboratory with the causative factor, it will be anybody's guess what's causing the disease.

DIAGNOSIS

Due to the fact that the signs and symptoms of Alzheimer's disease can be confused with many other neurological problems caused by many brain encephalopathy the only definite diagnosis is by microscopic examination of the brain after death.

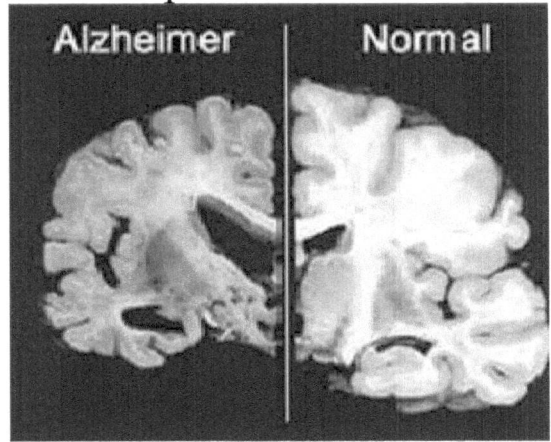

normal brain on the right side and abnormal atrophied brain on the left due to Alzheimer's desease.

The signs and symptoms of Alzheimer are

confusing with so many other conditions that have similar symptoms and it makes the diagnosis extremely difficult. I am sure there are many people that are mistakenly misdiagnosed as having the disease when in fact they do not have Alzheimer's but something else. Many other conditions can cause memory loss and be confused with Alzheimer's . Even with the latest technological diagnostic tools it is difficult to definitely diagnose dementia.

TREATMENTS

Treatments for dementia , senility and Alzheimer is experimental. there are several drugs used to treat Alzheimer's disease but there is no definite prove that the drugs actually help the patient. There are three drugs that are usually used to treat Alzheimer's patients, the donepezil, galantamine and Exelon. I have no idea how effective these drugs are and they have some side effects, such as vomiting, diarrhea, nausea, fatigue, insomnia, loss of appetite and weight loss . These side effects can have a detrimental effect on the patients health if taken over a prolong period of time. which makes you wonder if these drugs help the patients or hinder their recovery . This is something that the family doctor and the patients family should discuss in length what's the best for the patient

Since there is no definite cause and diagnosis for Alzheimer's disease, the doctors do their best with what they know and hope for the best. Researchers concluded that turmeric is an effective safe "drug" for the treatment of the behavioral and psychological symptoms of dementia in Alzheimer's patients.

Vitamins such as the B complex, B1, folic acid B9, C, calcium and magnesium and zinc help improve the memory.

Some foods that can boost the brain's memory are fatty fish, coffee, blueberries, turmeric, broccoli, pumpkin seeds, nuts and chocolate. A good nutrition is always good for anybody whether they have a memory loss or not. Besides prevention is better than any cure.

It is very important that patients with Alzheimer's , dementia and senility to have good sleep every night, good nutritional diet and regular exercises. This advice is good for anybody else too . Good nutrition and exercises is the best recipe for good health for everybody, no matter if they are one or 101 years old.

WHY DO PEOPLE GET SENILITY, DEMENTIA AND ALZHEIMER'S.

That's the million dollar question which unfortunately nobody has the answer. There are a lot of speculation of what causes this disease but nobody can really prove the real cause. As I said before, it is anybody's guess.
Senility, dementia and Alzheimer's are usually found in older people and can be due to many factors. As we all know the brain needs oxygen to survive like the rest of the body, so any interruption of fresh oxygen to the brain, even for a short period, will have an effect on the brain cells. One thing is for sure found in all Alzheimer's patients brain on microscopic examination. A shrunk brain full of plaques that killed the neurons in the brain. There are many theories what caused the plaques and the death of million of neurons, but they are still working to identify the real cause and find ways to prevent that from happening. Until then we all are waiting for that result.

ANY NUTRITIONAL CONNECTION TO SENILITY, dementia and Alzheimer's disease?

The fact that people in the island of Okinawa Japan that eat nutritional foods, work in their gardens everyday and remain healthy into very old age of 100 years old with few age related diseases including dementia, one can presume that indeed there is somewhere a connection that a good nutritional diet can stave off senility, dementia and Alzheimer's disease. The fact that there are some other places on earth that people with good diets and exercising daily like the Okinawa people have similar results as the Okinawa people, strongly suggest that indeed there is a connection between good nutritional diet and age related diseases.

Now it is up to the researchers, who already are contacting researches in those area to find exactly what's the connection between nutrition and senility and inform the rest of the people what to do to avoid the ravaging effects of senility and Alzheimer's disease. They already have an idea that a good nutritional diet and daily exercises help people stay healthy in their golden years. What their future suggestions will be, how to avoid dementia and other related diseases, it remains to be seen in the near future we hope. Maybe a nutritional pill for the elderly? We will see…

In the meantime, researchers are advising elderly people to eat a good nutritional diet, like the Mediterranean diet, exercising daily, sleep well at night and avoid dangerous substances that can cause damage to the brain.

I think that's a very good advise for all the people young and old. Following this advice the young will be preparing for their golden years and the elderly will be living their golden years.

LOW SALT DIET AND IODINE DEFICIENCY MAYBE CONFUSED WITH DEMENTIA AND ALZHEIMER'S.

A lot of people when they reach middle age and even earlier they have elevated blood pressure and when they go to their doctor they are advised to cut or eliminate their salt intake. This is a common advice for people with high blood pressure but the problem is that when they eliminate their salt intake it can create some body mineral deficiencies. Salt is an essential for nerve and muscle function and is needed for the regulation of the body fluids. If there is not enough salt intake, it can cause hyponatremia, an

extreme sodium deficiency that can cause serious health problems such as muscle cramps, nausea,, dizziness ,shock and even coma and death .
In chronic low salt intake it can cause iodine deficiency because salt is enriched with iodine to prevent hypothyroidism. Hypothyroidism is a condition where the thyroid gland does not produce enough thyroid hormones due to a lack of iodine in the people's diet. Many people get their iodine needs from the salt in their diet..
Hypothyroidism can mimic the symptoms of dementia with memory loss, fatigue and sensitive to heat and cold. So if the patient is on a low salt diet and has dementia symptoms, it might be a good idea for their doctors to check for hypothyroidism and other nutritional deficiencies. Older patients might not have a good balanced diet and develop all sorts of nutritional deficiencies and these deficiencies can mimic many diseases including dementia and Alzheimer's. So it is reasonable to expect from the family doctor to investigate all plausible causes before reaching a definite diagnosis and start unnecessary drug treatments for Alzheimer's which can have some severe side effects. But this is up to their doctor to do the necessary laboratory and other diagnostic tests before rushing into any drug treatments.

IODINE DEFICIENCY SIGNS AND SYMPTOMS
which mimic the Alzheimer's disease.

The readers might be wondering why I am writing about iodine deficiency when the book is about dementia and Alzheimer's.
The answer is simple. If dementia and Alzheimer's had unique clear cut signs and symptoms and could easily be diagnosed with laboratory and other diagnostic tests and not be confused with any other condition, I would not be writing about iodine deficiency. But the problem remains that Alzheimer's can mimic and be confused with many other conditions and the definite diagnosis is made only after death with the microscopic examination of the patient's brain.
One of the many conditions that can be confused with, is the iodine deficiency which causes hypothyroidism with symptoms mimicking Alzheimer's and that's why I write about iodine deficiency.
Iodine deficiency is a lack of the trace element iodine in the diet. Iodine is used by the body to produce thyroid hormones in the thyroid gland. Thyroid hormones are needed by the body to function properly. These hormones play a vital role in the regulation of various metabolic processes, particularly those involved in growth ,energy

expenditure , the body temperature, calcium balance, reproduction , muscle and nerve function. As we see iodine is a very important nutrient for the proper function of the thyroid gland which produces the thyroid hormones needed for the proper function of the whole body.

Symptoms of **hypothyroidism** are **Lethargy** and **tiredness**, muscular **weakness** and constant **fatigue**. Feeling cold even during the summer days, Difficulty concentrating, slowed mental processes , poor memory, and Depression.

Many of these symptoms are present in Alzheimer's' and dementia, so it is very important when the patient exhibits all these symptoms to rule out hypothyroidism caused by iodine deficiency or other nutritional deficiencies that cause similar symptoms.

With the iodine deficiency there is even a skin patch test you can do at home to see if you have iodine deficiency. You just put a few drops of iodine on your arm and see how long it will take to be absorbed by your skin and disappear. If you do not have iodine deficiency it will take more than 12 hours to be absorbed and disappear. If it disappears sooner it means your body needs iodine.

This is a crude test and it might not be reliable, so it is better to ask your doctor to check your iodine and thyroid hormone levels in a diagnostic laboratory.

The best way to supplement your diet with iodine is to eat foods that contain iodine, such as egg yolks, seafood, shrimps, foods and sea salt or iodized salt. But be careful not to overdo it with the salt as it can cause other problems in the body when you take too much.

.

DRUGS AFFECTING SHORT AND LONG TERM MEMORY LOSS

There are many prescription and non prescription drugs and foods or plants that can cause short and long term memory loss and can be confused with dementia and Alzheimer's .

Some of the drugs that affect memory are:
ant anxiety drugs such as Benzodiazepines, alprazolam (Xanax), chlordiazepoxide (Librium), etc.
Cholesterol Drugs (Statins) Examples: atorvastatin (Lipitor), fluvastatin (Lescol), lovastatin etc
Antidepressant Drugs (Tricyclic antidepressants) Examples: amitriptyline (Elavil), clomipramine etc
Hypertension Drugs (Beta-blockers) Examples: atenolol (Tenormin), carvedilol (Coreg), metoprolol etc
There also many opioids drugs, and other legal or illegal drugs that affect the human brain and its

functions.

Alcohol and tobacco can affect in a bad way the normal function of the brain.

It is always advisable to take into account all the plausible causes of memory loss when it happens and consult your health provider before you make any adjustments to any drug therapies you might have or jump into a premature diagnosis of dementia and Alzheimer's.

Retirement boredom and health risks

Many people are looking forwards to the day when they will end their working days and retire, get their pension and live their lives sitting around, enjoying their golden years without the worries of going to work for a living. Some people will adjust to their new routine sitting around without having to work for a living. some people will get bored without their working routing and they will start working part time to keep their time occupy. For others the boredom of the empty hours will cause mental and physical problems which can lead depression and anxieties.

All these factors can affect their appetite and their mood which can lead to nutritional deficiencies leading them to seek medical advice and prescription of drugs to treat these symptoms. Considering the above, it might be a good idea for people reaching retirement to plan ahead of time how they are going to spend all that free time they will have after their retirement. Perhaps they should ease into their retirement by cutting the amount of time they work gradually . This way they will have lots of time to organize their retirement better and it will not be an abrupt stop or their working time.

Anyway, everyone has a different way of planning and doing things including retirement and it is their own prerogative.

My 2cents advice is keep busy and keep moving, that's the only way to have a positive outlook in life. Besides when someone retires at age 65, they may have another twenty, thirty or even forty years of life, so it is important not think that because they retired from work that they retire from life too. Some people had very successful carriers after 65 and started successful business ,like Colonel Harland Sanders who is known for creating the world's fast-food chicken chain, Kentucky Fried Chicken.

OVERMEDICATIONS AND ABUSE OF ELDERLY PEOPLE IS A FACT HAPPENING EVERYDAY IN MANY PARTS OF THE WORLD.

The prospect of abuse and overmedicating the elderly people is real , exist and it does happens everyday. Over the years I watched on television documented abuses of elderly people suffering from Alzheimer's or other diseases. In one particular case a nurse killed a few elderly patients that were under her care. By the time she was caught she already killed six elderly patients.
In another case a caregiver was sexually abusing a patient with Alzheimer's and he was caught with a hidden camera placed by the patient's relatives.
In another case a woman caregiver was physically abusing her patient and she was also caught by a hidden camera placed by the patient's relatives that were concerned about the patient's unexplained bruises to his body.
In many cases elderly patients in geriatric institutions look like zombies from the many drugs that are taking everyday whether they need al those drugs or not. My guess is that with the medications the can control them easier .
Under normal conditions relatives and friends of those affected with Alzheimer's and dementia are concerned about their affliction and take good care

of them. However a few relatives might take advantage of their condition to abuse them mentally and even physically. Sometimes, even their own kids will take advantage of their parents memory loss to declare them mentally incompetent so that they have access to their parents assets for their own economic gain. This happens in rare occasions but still is happening. Unfortunately when the patient has a full blown case of Alzheimer's disease, there is nothing they can do about it. Their brain is not working anymore, their memory and reasoning is not working any more and it is a sad predicament they are in .

I am sure their doctors are doing everything possible to help their patients. However, due to the fact the Alzheimer's disease has no clear cause, diagnosis and treatment their doctors do not know which drugs work better for their condition and they might over prescribe medications for their patients which might have adverse side effects on their mood, appetite and health. Plus all the other medications that the patients already take for other conditions that they have , it creates a drug cocktail that might make the patients condition even worse .
I am sure the doctors have good intentions trying to help their patients but unfortunately they do not

have many choices due to the nature of the disease Alzheimer's.

With the advent of the internet many lonely elderly people both men and women are defrauded with the promise of love and marriage. As a result of this internet fraught many people end up penniless, depressed and even lonelier than before. In a few cases I watched on the Dr, Phil show, the fraudsters never met their victims in person; they only talked to them on the phone or texting and they always ask money from their victims. As sad as it may sounds , the victims were gullible enough to send their life savings to a stranger that they never met, just because the were promising love and asking for money. Anyway , that's what can happen when people are lonely and depressed .
That is why it very important to keep in touch with relatives and friends and seek advise when they are confronted with such situations.

HOW TO REDUCE THE RISK OF DEMENTIA AND ALZHEIMER'S.

Research is going on in many parts of the world to find the real cause of dementia and Alzheimer's. the research is mainly contacted in areas where the people live long time and they are healthy without dementia or Alzheimer's. a research in Japanese island Okinawa where people live over 100 years old , they are healthy and do not suffer from old age diseases , dementia, Alzheimer's and cardiovascular diseases. The research found that the people there live a simple life work in their gardens and the eat nutritional foods. One particular food which they consume in huge amounts every day is the purple sweet potatoes. Scientist found that the purple sweat potatoes is a powerhouse of nutrients especially anthocyanins which help to protect the brain and the cardiovascular system. Purple sweet potatoes are not found in many parts of the world but there are other foods that contain anthocyanins such as red and black grapes, black currants, blueberries, blackberries, red and blue cabbage.

The research also found that the people there, keep active all the time and they work in their gardens growing their own nutritional foods even when they are in their late nineties or even over 100 year olds. They also exercise in the marshal arts daily and it is not unusual to find people in their nineties to practice these defensive exercises.

The research is still going on trying to unravel the

mysteries of the longevity of the people living there with the hope to help other people in other parts of the world to achieve the same quality of life as the Okinawa people.

So far, one thing is clear, a simple life, keeping active and good nutrition promotes good health and longevity for the Japanese people that live there and perhaps other people might benefit from their habits.

Another research was done in England where elderly people keep busy organize tournaments of table tennis. People in their eighties and even nineties play completive table tennis games and they are in a very good state of health both physically and mentally. The people contacting the research wanted to know if walking was as good an exercise as completive table tennis. So they got people to volunteer in the research, dividing the volunteers in two groups, a walking group and a table tennis players. The researchers did all kind of medical tests including brain scans on the volunteers before and after a period of time. At the end of the research the tests and brain scans show a lot of improvements on both groups of volunteers. At the end of the research, All people reported that they felt better and some of them even reported that they had less anxieties and depression. The conclusion of the research was that exercises are very good at keeping the brain alert and avoid dementia and Alzheimer's.

Dr. Oz in one of his shows about Alzheimer's he said that some researchers discovered that when people breath through their nose it helps them with their memory. He even use the quote, "the nose knows" to emphasize that breathing through the nose is good for the brain and the memory.

SO WHAT DO THE EXPERTS RECOMMEND FOR REDUCING THE RISKS OF ALZHEIMER'S DISEASE.

According to several researches past and present on the people of Okinawa Japan , and other places they came to the conclusion that lifestyles matter. While nobody can change the people's genes, there are many risks factors that they can avoid. The daily habits can have an effect on people's life and dementia. At the present time there are no drugs or procedures that can cure or even effectively treat dementia. But people have the power to combat some of its major risk factors, including diabetes, high blood pressure, high cholesterol, stress, social isolation, and sleeplessness. The way people live today can have an effect on their health and the risk to get dementia in the future. The choices you make over the course of any average day , smoking, using drugs, poor diets leading to nutritional deficiencies, can determine whether you'll develop dementia years from now, as well as how quickly the disease will progress . So it is important to know the risks factors.

The risk factors are:

Smoking: several studies have linked smoking and mental decline raising the risk of dementia.

Smoking any type of smoke can influence your brain over a long period of time by depriving your body and your brain from fresh oxygen while you breath in the smoke of whatever you smoke. Some types of smoke are more harmful to the brain than others but the end result is that the smoke you inhale will affect your health sooner or later. There is even the suspicion that smoked meat and barbeque can cause dementia. So quit smoking while you are ahead of the game to protect your health and the risk of dementia.

High blood pressure:

People with high blood pressure over a prolong period of time will have a greater risk of developing dementia. High blood pressure affects the heart, the blood circulation and hardening of the arteries with a higher risk of a stroke , and developing dementia.

Keep your blood pressure in check.
It is advisable to control high blood pressure with diet, exercises, reduce your salt intake and if necessary the use of prescription drugs to regulate the blood pressure back to normal levels.

Diabetes:
people with type one and type two diabetes have an increased risk to develop dementia and cognitive impairment in their golden years. It is advisable to keep diabetes and blood sugar levels at normal range with good nutritional diets and exercises plus the recommended prescribed medications if needed.

High blood cholesterol levels:
High cholesterol levels is a risk factor for hypertension and cardiovascular disease and research has shown that people with these conditions have higher risk of developing dementia and Alzheimer's disease. It is important to keep the blood cholesterol levels within normal range with diet and exercises.

Alcohol
Alcohol is one of the most dangerous substance that causes many diseases such as cirrhosis of the liver cardiovascular disease, and brain intoxication. People that drink excessively have a higher risk of brain damage and dementia. Other

legal and illegal substances can cause damage to the brain leading to dementia.. It is advisable to reduce or eliminate the consumption of alcohol and other harmful substances to reduce the risk of dementia.

Head injuries:
People that had severe or repeated head injuries have greater risk to develop Alzheimer's disease due to damage to the brain. It is always a good idea to protect your head to avoid injuries whenever is possible. Athletes in contact sports have often head injuries and concussions and some of them developed Alzheimer's disease even before their golden years. Head injuries is a serious injury and If a head injury occur, seek medical treatment immediately. It is advisable to protect your head when you ride motorcycles and other activities that have the potential of a head injury.

Some other medical conditions can increase the risk of developing dementia. These conditions are , Parkinson's disease, down's syndrome and some learning disabilities.

Some researches suggest that even a low level of education is a risk for Alzheimer's disease. A research done with nuns that usually have a clean living found that they had less risk of dementia than other groups of people. Nuns that had lower level of education they were more prone to develop dementia. They also found that the greater their education the better their cognitive abilities in the tests. . Education and past experiences help people to prevent Alzheimer's disease. Benefits of education is that exercising the brain , protects it in the long run from dementia. Brain exercises are good for the young and the old.

Some researches also suggest to avoid fried foods and foods high in saturated fat to protect the cardiovascular system and the brain from dementia. We know that these foods are not good for your health, so it is a good idea to avoid them.

They also suggest that people should sleep seven to ten hours every night. It is advisable to have regular hours of sleep every night not to disturb the internal clock of the body and brain.

The above are among the many risks factors to avoid for a better health and minimize the chances of suffering from dementia.

Researchers recommend a healthy living to prevent dementia in the golden years.

Researchers also recommend what people should do to improve their chances of not getting Alzheimer's disease.

1) KEEP ACTIVE, KEEP MOVING.

Number one on their list is to keep moving, the healthier your body is, the healthier brain can be. Their study In Okinawa Japan, where people exercise daily they have fewer health problems with less memory loss. Elderly people there are socially connected to society and highly respected and this stave off dementia. That is something that people can learn from and perform in their daily life to accomplish the same results as the Japanese do.

A research study done in England with two groups of elderly people with one group exercising with a brisk walking an hour a day for 10 weeks and the other elderly group playing competitive table tennis for an hour a day for ten weeks.
After 10 weeks brisk walking, and table tennis, both groups had better cognitive abilities, Due to more aerobic activities. Their brain scans showed that they even have thicker cortex. Regular exercises reduces anxiety as well. So keep moving and you will be healthier and decrease the risk of dementia too.

2) GOOD NUTRITIONAL HABITS.

Eat a healthy nutritional diet like the Mediterranean diet. The food you eat provides the fuel for your body and brain and the

Mediterranean diet provides the best nutrition. The Mediterranean Greeks used to say " νους υγιης εν σοματι υγιη», which means " a healthy mind in a healthy body". In this diet includes such things as whole grains, leafy green vegetables, nuts, fish, berries, olive oil, beans, as well as limited amounts of cheese and meat. The goal of this diet is to control your weight, blood pressure, blood sugar and reduce the risk of cardiovascular disease. It was also found to reduce the risk of Alzheimer's up to 50 percent. The people of Okinawa Japan eat a lot Sweet potatoes which also protect the cardiovascular system from disease.

3) Cut down your fat intake.
Reduce or eliminate the saturated fat completely and replace it with healthy olive oil. Saturated fat damages the blood vessels causing arteriosclerosis which is a risk factor for the brain and dementia. Olive oil helps protect the cardiovascular system from arteriosclerosis and might prevent strokes and memory loss.

4) Never stop learning .Keep learning throughout your life .
Learning new things stimulates your brain to work better and it is an exercise for your brain and mind forcing your brain to sharpen different cognitive

processes including attention and memory.
Learning a new language or a new instrument helps the brain to
Boost memory with focusing and keep attention concentration.
 The Benefits from brain exercises helps ward off dementia and Alzheimer's. so keep learning new things everyday to sharpen your brain and avoid dementia. The old adage " use it or loose" is apparently valid for the brain too.

Researchers also found that electrical stimulation of the brain, Increases the attention span and Can help older people have better memory, but this is still in the experimental stage .

5) Grow a garden.
If you live in a house and you have enough room in your backyard to grow your own garden , it will be a great idea to grow your own garden for the good of your body and mind. Working in the garden planting the vegetables you like for your own consumption is a great feeling to see the rewards of your efforts. The physical work is a great exercise for your body and a serene feeling for your mind. In other words you kill two birds with one stone, exercising your body and the tranquility of your mind.
When your planting gives fruition you will have

good nutritional vegetables to enjoy for your family and even share some with your friends or neighbors. The physical work strengthens muscles in your hands, arms, shoulders, back, and it is a good exercise for your brain too. Of course go easy at the beginning and do not overdo it. It is a very good idea to use an elastic support for your back and knee pads to protect your knees when kneeling.

Gardening takes your mind off the daily qualms and it fights off anxieties and depression. So keep gardening for the good of your body and your mind. Researchers found that is the secret of the people of Okinawa Japan for their longevity, good health and less dementia.

6) Dance the night away.

Whenever you have the chance get up and dance. Dancing is one of the best exercises for the body and the mind. You do not have to be a good dancer to enjoy dancing, just walk to the music beat with your partner. You can have lots of fun dancing while strengthening your bones and muscles, and improving your posture and balance . Studies found that dancing with a group or a partner you are exercising social smarts which is beneficial for your brain and memory. Dancing will take your mind off the daily worries and you will have lots of fun which is good for your mind to fend off anxieties and depression. Anxiety and depression can be a symptom of dementia and with dancing you take your mind of any anxieties you might have……..

7) GET A DOG AND WALK DAILY.
The doc will keep you good company and an excuse to exercise walking your dog daily.
if you have a dog join or form a dog walking group to expand your social network. Socializing with other people is good for your brain and memory to fight off dementia.

8) JOIN A LAUGHTER CLUB OR WATCH FUNNY VIDEOS.
There is a saying that " laughter is the best medicine" and a new research suggests that humor can improve short-term memory in older adults.. Humor increases endorphins sending dopamine to the brain providing a sense of pleasure . Laughing daily will improve the quality of your life. So it is a good idea to join a laughter club and have lots of laughing time with old and new friends. That will make your life better and will ward off anxiety, depression and dementia. Some years ago, I was reading in the newspaper that a doctor gave his depressed patient a prescription for laughter with the reasoning that the laughter is the best medicine.

9) spend time with younger people.

There was a 90 year surgeon that he was still working and teaching younger doctors his surgical expertise, and when a reporter ask him why he was still working, his answer was'' working with younger people makes me feel young".

Research found that elderly people working with young people as mentors have better physical health and better memory. I guess it is like growing a garden, you get the satisfaction of seeing young people growing up and thriving with your guidance. If you have young kids, grandkids and great grandkids, it is a good idea to spend time with them and even play with them at times. It will make you feel younger again and you will have the chance to teach them your life long experiences and expertise. That will help keep you active both physically and mentally and it is a lot better than sitting in an institution for the elderly or watching television.

Recent and ongoing experimental researches explore the possibilities of using blood plasma from younger people to older people to rejuvenate the brain. Experiments on animals and human volunteers showed promising results.

Older Volunteers had blood plasma from younger people and got better in their brain functions. The question remains if this is some form of the Frankenstein experiments or Is it the fountain of youth that will transform the treatment of Alzheimer's patients.
Time will tell…
 In the United States of America, doctors opened medical clinics offering young blood transfusions for $8000-10,000. But the FDA did not approve that and the clinics were closed.
The idea of blood or plasma transfusion for rejuvenation and strength is not really new. Some completive Olympic athletes were using that process for strength and endurance. I am not sure if the Olympic organizers still allow such a practice or if they banned it.

If you are caring for parents or relatives with Alzheimer's:

If you made the sacrifice to take care of your parents in their difficult times, I commend you for that. Your parents did everything they could to raise you and from your actions seems that they did a good job. Your job is hard and difficult but at least you know that your parents are in good hands, your caring hands.
They are not abandon in an elderly peoples institution where there is no privacy and sometimes the care is mediocre, and sometimes they are abused both mentally and physically by indifferent staff or other inmates. Your parents are in the caring hands of their loved ones, your hands, and even though their mental capacity is gone, if you look in their eyes you will clearly see that they are appreciate your efforts and they proud of you.
Do whatever you can to make their final years

comfortable and if you can afford it, get some help to help you care for your loved ones.

Do not forget to take care of yourself too, you have to be strong and healthy so that you can take care of others.

In my book :
EAT THE RIGHT FOODS
FOR OPTIMUM HEALTH :
Available at amazon.com

In that book I describe the best nutritional foods for optimum health for everyone even for people that have symptoms of Alzheimer's. If you and the parents you take care off, eat the nutritional foods your bodies need you will both benefit. if your parents have been misdiagnosed and they do not have the deadly disease but suffer from nutritional deficiencies which can mimic the symptoms of dementia, they will have a good chance their condition to improve , even get healthy again.

In the meantime take good care of them and yourself.

Spend time with them, talk to them, cook them nutritional foods, take them for a walk, help them plant a garden, tell them a joke even though they will probably forget what you were telling them in 5 minutes. it makes their life more livable and comfortable. It is a lot better than living isolated, lonely and depressed in an elderly institution.

Follow the doctors recommendations and the experts recommendations in this book to make their lives more comfortable . Ask the doctor to recommend some vitamins and minerals for them, that might help correct any nutritional deficiency. And maybe just maybe someday in the near future the scientist will find the cure for this disease and your parents will be well again and grateful that you were there and took good care of them in their time of need. If the cure never comes before they are gone forever, at least you will have the satisfaction that you did everything you could to make their last days comfortable.

.

CONCLUSION

There is no question that there are many people that have the deadly Alzheimer's encephalopathy and sadly their lives are destroyed by the ravaging effects of the disease. However there are many people that do not have the deadly disease and wrongly are diagnosed and treated as Alzheimer's patients because they have similar symptoms to Alzheimer's disease. One thing is certain that people should eat a good nutritional balanced diet and exercise daily to keep their bodies in optimum health. By doing that their bodies will function properly and they might have a good chance to avoid or at least delay the ravaging effects Alzheimer's disease.
Until the researchers and scientist find out what really causes dementia and the proper treatment, all the people young and especially the old should follow the healthy lifestyle of the people of Okinawa and the Mediterranean diet. Keep active exercising and good nutritional diet will safeguard you health and you will have a good chance to avoid the ravaging effects of Alzheimer's disease. There are no guarantees in life but if you take good care of your body and mind you might have a chance to live to the ripe age of 100 years old ,like the Okinawa people in Japan with your mental capacities intact! I think it is a chance

worth taking, taking care of yourself, which is priority number one for all living organisms.

EPILOG

Alzheimer's and other deadly diseases are ruining the lives of many people in all parts of the world turning their golden years into wasted years. People that once were healthy and vibrant Are turned into zombies unable to care for themselves or even recognize their loved ones. Alzheimer's is the disease that most people reaching their golden years are afraid of. The prospect of loosing your memory and unable to take care of yourself is extremely frightening. Unfortunately nobody knows exactly what is the cause of this deadly disease and there is no known effective treatment for a cure. Scientist all over the world are working hard to find the cause and cure for Alzheimer's. So far their research identified the risk factors of the disease and it is a good idea to avoid these risky factors with the hope that will help to prevent the development of dementia. They also identified that people in certain parts of the world do not have many health issues and dementia due to their healthy lifestyles. The lifestyles of those people in Okinawa Japan and the other areas with similar lifestyles that for some reason are protected from memory loss and dementia is simple. They keep busy working in their gardens, exercising daily and they have a healthy nutritional diet.

So, until the mystery of the cause of this disease is solved and a definite cure is found, it is prudent to follow the lifestyles of those people that already seem to be immune to dementia. It is also prudent to follow the recommendations of the experts to keep moving, exercising and have a healthy nutritional diet to stave off memory loss and dementia.

Book description.

Alzheimer's is a degenerating and progressive brain disorder that slowly destroys memory and thinking skills, and eventually the ability to carry out the simplest tasks. The patients afflicted with this condition eventually become completely incapacitated .
This book describes the risk factors of Alzheimer's and how to avoid those risks.
In this book you will find how the lifestyle of some people in certain countries affect their life positively and they have no health issues or dementia and they live well over 100 years old.
In this book, you will find the recommendations of many experts how to delay or even stave off dementia.
If you want to know how to prepare for your golden years and have a good chance to avoid the worst type of dementia , Alzheimer's, this book is for you.
If you want to know how to care for your loved ones when they are afflicted with dementia, you

will find useful suggestions in this book.

www.ingramcontent.com/pod-product-compliance
Lightning Source LLC
Chambersburg PA
CBHW030734180526
45157CB00008BA/3164